The Tincture-Maker's Cheat-Sheet:
A pocket reference for tincture-makers and herbalists

© 2017 Dafydd Monks

The moral rights of the author have been asserted.

All rights reserved. No part of this publication may be reproduced, distributed, or transmitted in any form or by any means, including photocopying, recording, or other electronic or mechanical methods, without the prior written permission of the publisher, except in the case of brief quotations embodied in critical reviews and certain other non-commercial uses permitted by copyright law. For permission requests, write to the publisher at the email address below.

All Enquiries to herbs@sbm-cymru.co.uk

Second Edition, 2017.

Published by Snowdonia Botanical Medicine, Caernarfon, Wales

Typeset in Swansea.

ISBN 978-1979500784

Printed by CreateSpace, an Amazon.com Company.

The Tincture-Maker's Cheat-Sheet

A pocket reference for tincture-makers and herbalists

By

Dafydd R Ll Monks BSc (Hons.)

http://www.sbm-cymru.co.uk

http://www.herbary.co.uk

Dedicated to all those who have helped me along this path, but in particular to Robyn James, mistress of numbers and herbalist extraordinaire without whose teaching this book would not be possible…

Contents

Part 1: Introduction

Introduction	p.1
What is a Tincture?	p.2
Why Should I Make my Own?	p.3
What Equipment do I need?	p.4
Understanding a Tincture	p.6
Ethanol, Grain Spirit, Vodka	p.7
Maceration: Your First Tincture	p.9
Bottling, Labeling, Recording	p.11
Fresh Tinctures	p.12
Advanced Tincturemaking	p.13
Ethanolic Glycerites	p.17
How to Use This Book	p.18

Part 2: The Formulary

List of herbs and suggested specs/methods	p.21

Part 3: The Cheat Sheets

Tincture-making with Vodka Data Tables	p.41
Tincture-making with Ethanol Dried Herb Data Tables	p.50
Tincture-making with Ethanol Fresh Herb Data Tables	p.80

Part 4: Appendices

Schedule III/20 Tincture Specs	p.95
UK Law on Tincture Making	p.96
Further Reading	p.98
Suppliers	p.99
Glossary	p.101
Measurement Conversion Table	p.103

Introduction

If you do not know what a tincture is, this book is very likely not for you. However, I'm very much hoping that you, the reader, are a herbalist or pharmacist— whether practicing clinically, making herbal remedies for family health, or are just interested in the process of preserving medicinal plants as alcoholic extracts.

This book is not a comprehensive resource on making medicines — it aims only to cover the process of making tinctures as used in Western Herbal Medicine. What it will do is simplify that process for those who already use tinctures and would like to make their own. It is a reference for understanding how tinctures are made, the mathematics involved, and other considerations in making your own medicinal tinctures of good quality and medicinal effect.

My background is originally in the aviation industry, and there, we have various little books of data tables that simplify the mathematics of tasks into an easy to access form and speed up those tasks. I thought that the mathematics of tincture-making could do with the same kind of treatment: The main portion of this book is a set of data-tables that you can use quickly and easily to work out the appropriate quantities of ingredients to make tinctures of a given specification. Hence the title: 'The Tincture-Maker's Cheat Sheet'.

What is a Tincture?

A tincture is an alcoholic extract of a medicinal plant. The alcohol serves two functions: Extraction and Preservation. The alcohol used in tincture making, ethanol, is a very useful solvent as it has two very important qualities. It is completely miscible (dissolvable in water) and due to its structure* it is amphipathic; dissolving both hydrophilic (water soluble) and hydrophobic (oil soluble) plant constituents, as well as resins and gums which are not readily soluble in water. Alcohol is also a good preservative: when alcohol concentrations in tinctures exceed about 20% by volume biological decomposition is slowed, and at high concentrations may be halted altogether as evinced by medical specimen collections which, before the discovery of formaldehyde used to be pickled in ethanol.

Alcohol has been used to preserve medicines for a long time. The distillation of alcohol was discovered by the Arab chemist Al-Kindi in 9th Century Iraq, although there is evidence of the use of stills as far back as ancient Egypt. Originally the distilled spirit that first gushed from the stills of the medieval Arab and Persian chemists was used for extracting and preserving medicines. The introduction of distillation to the Western world in

---
* An alcohol molecule consists of a carbon chain (always nonpolar) and a OH group (which is polar)

the late medieval period coincided with the rise of the apothecaries as producers and distributors of medicines, and it is to them that we must owe the introduction of alcoholic tinctures to both conventional pharmacy, and as the apothecaries' techniques (and use of plant-based medicines) passed from modern pharmaceutical practice, modern herbal medicine.

Why Should I Make My Own?

A suitable answer to this question is 'why not'. Although a somewhat flippant answer, the multitude of reasons for making your own tinctures are beyond the scope of this book. I would however leave you with a few points to think on:

Making your own tinctures is empowering. It is a declaration of independence in the practice of herbal medicine, removing a dependence on large suppliers. It protects us should our access to tinctures be removed. It also keeps us using, practicing and developing pharmacy skills that many will have only tried while training. You can use your own plant material to make your tinctures — herbs that you have grown and foraged yourself.

You can be sure of the quality. You know what all the inputs to your tincture were, and you can judge the quality of the product you make with your own senses to verify its quality.

Lastly, satisfaction. It is satisfying to make your own medicines knowing that you have created them from leaf and root through to finished product.

What Equipment Do I Need?

My suggestion for the kind of set up you need to make pretty much any of the tinctures in this book (with the exception of distilled tinctures or percolated fluid extracts) is:

- A set of digital scales with 1g resolution
- 1 or 2 2-4 litre pans
- Large (clean) wooden spoon
- Glass beakers: 500 ml and 1L capacity, alternatively; Pyrex measuring jugs
- Conical flasks: 500 ml and 1L capacity, alternatively; clean bottles will suffice
- A sieve
- A large funnel
- 10-micron filter paper, alternatively coffee filters
- Large, clean 'Kilner' jars with rubber seals

* Clean bottles to contain the finished product.
* A large piece of muslin, clean pillow case, or tincture press.

Most kitchenware shops or hardware shops should stock these items, and they are certainly all available cheaply on Amazon. Amazon can be a very good source of cheap laboratory grade glassware — a set of measuring beakers and conical flasks will set you back about £20.

To distil *hydrolats* (mixtures of un-separated floral waters and essential oils), you will need an alembic still, some rubber tubing, and a small electrical water pump.

Some fluid extracts are made in a device called a percolator which is a column containing the *marc* - the *menstruum* drips through the marc giving a finished tincture in as little as a couple of days.

For more information on buying an alembic still or percolation column see the appendices.

Understanding a Tincture Spec.

Look at any bottle of tincture on your dispensary shelf, and you will notice it has a specification on its label that looks something like this:

Crataegus monogyna Flos. 1:3 25% Fresh Herb Tincture

This is an example of the label on a bottle of Hawthorne blossom tincture. The Latin name and 'flos' should be self-apparent if you are working with herbs already. The 1:3 bit is the strength specification: it means that the ratio of herb material (Known as the *Marc*) to the *Menstruum*, or liquid that the tincture was made with is one part of herb to three parts of liquid.

If you look at a medicinal pharmaceutical liquid, be it a tincture or eye drops from your local chemist, you may notice letters after the strength specification; w/w, w/v, v/v or v/w. The W means 'weight', and the 'V' means volume. Due to the pragmatic nature of tincturing herbs, which are solid, our tinctures will be w/v or weight in volume tinctures. Thus a 1:3 w/v tincture will contain one gram of *marc* or herb material to every three millilitres of *menstruum* or liquid.

The 25% refers to the amount of alcohol the tincture contains as a percentage of the liquid. I.E.:

Alcohol by volume. It is exactly the same as the alcohol spec. of your bottle of wine or tin of beer.

To complicate matters, tinctures can be made to either a start-spec or an end-spec. The start-spec is the ratio of *menstruum* added to the *marc* at the start of the process; the end-spec is the ratio of herb to the amount of *menstuum* expressed *from* the marc at the end of the process. Many tincture-makers use the start-spec, though it is handy to also know your end spec, and yield. To calculate yield, divide the amount of expressed *menstruum* from your tincture by the total amount of *menstruum you you started with.*

Discussing the merits of which specification or technique to use to best extract what constituent in which tincture is beyond the scope of this book. I have given some examples to follow in part 2; however these are very much starting points for you to work from as you experiment and begin to learn what methods work best for you and your herbs.

Ethanol, Grain Spirit, Vodka

Perhaps the most important element of your tincture, apart from the herbal material you are extracting is the solvent you are using; your alcohol. Although many people refer to ethanol and grain spirit as one and the same, pure ethanol is hard to make and very hard to come by, due to ethanol forming an azeotrope with water. This means that when ethanol and water are boiled, at roughly 96% ethanol content, the vapour leaving the still is identical to what is being boiled in the still pot. The azeotrope is 95.63% ethanol and 4.37% water (by weight). Ethanol boils at 78.4°C, water boils at 100°C, but the azeotrope boils at 78.2°C, which is lower than either of its constituents: in practice no further distillation can take place. So the 'purest ethanol' you are likely to encounter is 96% grain spirit. I like HaymanKimia's (Soil association certified) Grain Spirit 96% BP. It is ideally suited to making tinctures.

Many sources on making tinctures consider the use of 96% grain spirit to be equivalent to 100% ethanol, and to all intents and purposes it is, however if you are as pedantic as I am, you may like to account for the 4% in the specification of your tincture. If you consider 96% Grain Spirit to be 'pure alcohol' your specifications will be out by a small percent.

Tincture Specifications 100% Ethanol & 96% Grain Spirit:

Spec: Using 100% Ethanol	Actual Spec: Using 96% Grain Spirit
25%	24%
45%	43.20%
60%	57.60%
90%	86.40%

As you can see, the discrepancy between our theoretically 100% ethanol and our actual 96% grain spirit is negligible enough to not affect our tincture's shelf life or extraction of constituents. However the difference is worth knowing about — if nothing else than for use in a herbalist's pub quiz!

If you do not have access to strong spirit, you can use vodka or a similar 35% - 40% spirit to make your tinctures. These tinctures will be limited in strength — you won't be able to make anything stronger than a 40% dried herb tincture, or a 30% fresh herb tincture, and you will be limited to maceration, however you can still make satisfactory macerated tinctures of good quality using vodka.

Maceration: Your First Tincture

Historically, most tinctures made by the apothecaries were macerations of dried herbs. This means that dried herb material was soaked in alcohol and then expressed after some time. This will serve as a good example of making your first tincture. Dried-herb, macerated tinctures were traditionally 1:5s, though it is possible to make 1:3s, especially for roots, berries and barks. For an example of a maceration, let's look at a tincture of Valerian Root *Valeriana officinalis radix* 1:3 45%. Place a kilogram of finely chopped, dried valerian root in your 'Kilner' jar or clip-top bucket; add 1.35 litres of grain spirit, and 1.65 litres of water. Poke down the roots to ensure that as little as possible is exposed to the air, and store in a dark place for 6 weeks before expressing.

Some sources suggest shaking or stirring your tincture while it is macerating, some sources leave it well alone until it is ready to express. I tend to leave mine undisturbed.

If you have springy herb material that refuses to stay submerged in the *menstruum*, marbles are your friend: Get some heavy marbles, sterilise them and place them on top of your *marc* to keep it submerged.

After the maceration jar has sat for its required duration, it will be time to express the *menstruum* from the *marc*. You can either tip your *marc* into a piece of muslin or clean pillow-case for larger batches, and let the *menstruum* drip out before squeezing thoroughly, or you can invest in a tincture press to give mechanical assistance to expression. Some herbs will give a very high yield of expressed *menstruum* indeed - especially fruits and berries. Some, such as dried foliage will not give as great a yield.

Bottling, Labeling, Recording

I recommend that you filter your expressed tincture before bottling. This is especially true of dry-herb tinctures, which are prone to have lots of 'bits' and 'silt' at the bottom of the maceration vessel.

Place a large coffee filter, or folded filter paper (fold round filter-papers into 4, making a triangle and open up one side to form a cone) into a funnel and filter your newly made tincture. Pass the tincture through this filter taking care not to over-fill the paper, allowing sediment to pass. However, some thick mucilaginous tinctures like *Althea officinalis Radix* will not filter well through paper and are best filtered through cloth only.

Label your storage bottles with the tincture's Latin and English names, full spec/strength, date of manufacture and a batch number. This information should also be recorded in a notebook or electronic record.

Devote a notebook page to each tincture you make including the source of the herb material/date it was collected or bought, the Latin and English names, full spec/strength, date of manufacture, batch number and amounts of herb material, grain spirit, and other liquid added to the tincture. This is your protection should anything unfortunate happen with your tincture - you have appropriately documented what you did.

Batch numbers are important - some people suggest a plain serial number, the only problem with this is that a long batch number is not memorable. My suggestion would be to use the following format

1758

This is actually the batch number of the last tincture I made. The first two digits are the year - 2017. The second digits are a short serial number, signifying that it is the 58th tincture I made in 2017. This keeps your batch numbers simple and record-keeping easy

Fresh Tinctures

Which works best? A tincture made with dried herbs or fresh? In theory, dried herbs weigh a lot less than fresh herb, so a tincture made with dried herbs will be stronger as more herbal material has gone into it. However, some practitioners like tinctures made with fresh herbs. The plant material is in a closer state to the growing plant and will be less likely to have lost volatile constituents.

Because they are fresh, some consider tinctures made with fresh herbs to be more 'vital' in nature than dried tinctures. In many ways there is little difference between making a tincture with dried or fresh herbs. The only real difference is that fresh plant material is 70% - 80% water by weight. This latent water must be accounted for to ensure that there is sufficient alcohol to preserve your tincture or extract the desired constituents. In practice, multiply the weight of your herb by .75 and deduct the result (in millilitres) from the amount of water you add to your tincture. Or use the fresh herb tables in this book (which have the latent water accounted for in the amounts of *menstruum* used and the alcohol-water ratio).

Advanced Tincture-making

So, you've tried making some macerated tinctures, and you quite like them, but part of you wishes you could make something a little stronger. Fear not. You can. When you make a tincture with grain spirit and water, you are effectively making your own vodka of a desired strength to use as a solvent in your tincture. What a waste. What if the water 'phase' of your tincture was a strong infusion, decoction or floral water/*hydrolat*? It would make your tincture considerably stronger, and extract a much fuller range of constituents. If you infuse, decoct or distil half of your *marc* you can easily attain a 1:1 tincture for most roots, barks, and berries and a 1:2 tincture for foliage, flowers or blossoms. These tinctures are in a way hybrid macerations: half the marc is still macerated, but the half that is processed will give an extraction that is much more suited to the type of plant material you are extracting than a plain maceration!

Fluid Extracts

'Fluid Extracts' are strong tinctures with a 1:1 specification. The name is confusing, as all tinctures are extracts in fluid. Fluid extracts require the use of a percolation column. It is beyond the scope of this handbook to describe percolation but use the 1:1 tables with your percolation column if you have access to one.

Infused Tinctures

These are best suited to non-volatile flowers, foliage or berries. Place half your *marc* in a glass bowl or pan and cover with boiling water. Use about 1 ½ times as much water as you will need in making your tincture as the plant material will absorb some of the water. Strain off the infusion and add to the other half of the *marc* in your maceration pot in place of water.

Decocted Tinctures

Woody roots, rhizomes and barks often need decocting, or boiling to break down the plant material and extract the active constituents. Take half your *marc*, place in a pan; add double the amount of water you need for your maceration and bring to the boil. Simmer for 15 minutes or until the volume of water has reduced by half; whichever occurs first. Strain the decoction through a sieve, measure, and add to the other half of the *marc* in your maceration pot in place of water. If you find you are a bit short, you can add a bit of cold water to the decoction to make the volume back up to the required amount.

Distilled Tinctures

If you have access to an alembic still, or other ways of producing or acquiring floral waters or *hydrolats* you absolutely must use them in tincture making. Needless to say, aromatic flowers, blossoms, and leaves respond best to distillation — there is no point distilling a herb that is not aromatic or fragrant. However the extraction of volatile constituents is significantly improved by distillation and will result in a lovely, aromatic tincture. Place half your *marc* in your still, add double to three times the amount of water you aim to use in your tincture and light the still. Distil until you have the amount of floral water you need for your tincture, then add this to your maceration pot in place of ordinary water.

Calculating Water

There is not enough space in the book to devote separate cheat sheets for the 'two step' tinctures. If you are making an infused, decocted or distilled fresh herb tincture, half of your plant material will not be macerated, and thus won't add to the total water content of the tincture. For the sake of accuracy, add together the amount of added water from the dried and fresh cheat sheets of the same spec and divide by 2 - this will give you the amount of infusion, decoction or distillate required for your 'advanced' 2-step tincture

Ethanolic Glycerites

Somewhere between a tincture and a glycerite, ethanolic glycerites are preparations that contain both alcohol and glycerine. Often such extractions are simple macerations, with the *menstruum* being a mix of grain spirit and glycerine. The two ratios that are typically used are 70% glycerine to 30% grain spirit, or 50%:50%. Macerate for 6 weeks and express. The grain spirit preserves the glycerine which is otherwise wont to spoil unless refrigerated. These preparations extract aromatic constituents well, and taste nice due to the sweetness of the glycerine. You absolutely must try making a Damask Rose ethanolic glycerite. Seriously, do it… …and tell me it's not amazingly lovely!

How to Use This Book

This book is divided into two sets of tables.

Firstly there is a list of tinctures, with suggested strength and alcohol specs., along with a list of suitable methods to make them. These are just suggestions - the beauty of making your own tinctures is that you have the freedom to vary from these suggestions and make exactly what you want, or have enough herb or alcohol to make.

Secondly, and more important, are the amount tables - the 'cheat sheets'. These will take the calculating out of your tincture-making. They are organised primarily by alcohol content, subdivided by strength of tincture. There is a different value table for each strength and alcohol content of tincture, and separate tables for dried and fresh plant material. I have also included tables for 1:3 fresh herb and 1:5 and 1:3 dried herb vodka tinctures.

In order not to be pedantically silly, amounts on the cheat sheets are rounded to the nearest millilitre for measurements given in ml, and litres are rounded to 2 decimal places - accurate to 5 ml per litre in quantities above 1 litre.

The information is this book is believed to be accurate and is provided in good faith, however the author accepts no liability for any injury, loss or damage caused or incurred from the use of this data. You are advised to double check these calculations yourself if you have any doubts as to their accuracy or suitability.

Part 2

The Formulary:

A list of suggested tinctures

The Formulary: Suggested Strength,

Latin Name	English Name
Achillea millefolium Herba	Yarrow Herb
Aconitum nepellus Herba	Aconite Herb
Acorus calamus Rad.	Sweet Flag Root
Aesculus hippocastanum Sem.	Horse Chestnut Seed
Agrimonia eupatoria Herba	Agrimony Herb
Agropyron repens Rad.	Couchgrass Rhizome
Alchemilla arvensis Herba	Parsley Piert Herb
Alchemilla vulgaris Herba	Ladies Mantle Herb
Allium sativum	Garlic Bulb
Althaea officinalis Fol.	Marshmallow Leaf
Althaea officinalis Rad.	Marshmallow Root
Anemone pulsatilla Herba	Pasque Flower Herb
Angelica archangelica Herba	Angelica Herb
Angelica archangelica Rad.	Angelica Root
Angelica sinensis Rad.	Dong quai Root
Anthemis nobilis Flos.	Chamomile Flowers
Apium graveolens Sem.	Celery Seed
Arcostaphylos uva-ursi Fol.	Bearberry Leaf
Arctium lappa Rad.	Burdock Root

Alcohol & Tincturemaking Processes

Strength	% Alcohol	Suggested Process Type(s)
1:5, 1:3, 1:1	25%, 45%	Distilled, Infused, Macerated
1:3	70%	Macerated
1:5, 1:3	60%	Macerated
1:3, 1:1	25%	Decocted, Macerated
1:5, 1:3	25%, 45%	Infused, Macerated
1:5, 1:3, 1:1	25%, 45%	Decocted, Macerated
1:5, 1:3	25%	Infused, Macerated
1:5, 1:3, 1:1	25%	Infused, Macerated
1:2, 1:1	45%	Macerated
1:5, 1:3	25%	Infused, Macerated
1:3, 1:1	25%	Macerated
1:3, 1:1	25%, 45%	Infused, Macerated
1:5, 1:3	35%, 45%	Distilled, Decocted, Macerated
1:3, 1:1	35%, 45%	Distilled, Decocted, Macerated
1:3	25%, 45%	Decocted, Macerated
1:3, 1:1	25%, 45%	Distilled, Infused, Macerated
1:3, 1:1	70%	Macerated
1:3	25%	Infused, Macerated
1:3, 1:1	25%, 45%	Decocted, Macerated

The Formulary: Suggested Strength,

Latin Name	English Name
Arnica montana Flos.	Arnica Flower
Artemisia absinthium Herba	Wormwood Herb
Artemisia vulgaris Herba	Mugwort Herb
Astralagus membranaceus Rad.	Astragalus Root
Avena sativa Sem.	Oat Seed
Ballota nigra Herba	Black Horehound Herb
Baptisia tinctoria Rad.	Wild Indigo Root
Barosma betulina Fol.	Buchu Leaf
Berberis aquifolium Rad.	Oregon Grape Root
Berberis vulgaris Cort.	Barberry Bark
Betula alba Fol.	Birch Leaf
Borago officinalis Herba	Borage Herb
Calendula officinalis Flos.	Marigold Flowers 25%
Calendula officinalis Flos.	Marigold Flowers 90%
Capsella bursa-pastoris Herba	Shepherds Purse Herb
Capsicum minimum Fruct.	Cayenne Pepper
Carduus marianus Sem.	Milk Thistle Seed
Cassia angustifolia	Senna Pods
Caulophylum thalictroides Rad.	Blue Cohosh Root

Alcohol & Tincturemaking Processes

Strength	% Alcohol	Suggested Process Type(s)
1:8	35%	Infused, Macerated
1:3, 1:1	35%, 45%	Infused, Macerated
1:3, 1:1	25%, 45%	Infused, Macerated
1:3, 1:1	25%	Decocted, Macerated
1:3, 1:1	25%	Macerated
1:3, 1:1	25%, 45%	Infused, Macerated
1:3	25%, 60%	Decocted, Macerated
1:3	45%, 60%	Distilled, Infused, Macerated
1:3	35%, 45%	Decocted, Macerated
1:3	35%	Decocted, Macerated
1:3	25%, 45%	Infused, Macerated
1:3	25%, 45%	Infused, Macerated
1:3	25%	Macerated
1:3, 1:1	90%	Macerated
1:3	25%, 45%	Infused, Macerated
1:3	70%	Macerated
1:3, 1:1	45%	Decocted, Macerated
1:3	35%	Infused, Macerated
1:3	35%, 70%	Decocted, Macerated

The Formulary: Suggested Strength,

Latin Name	English Name
Centella asiatica Herba	Gotu Kola Herb
Centraria islandica	Iceland Moss
Chamaelirium luteum Rad.	False Unicorn Root
Chionanthus virginicus Cort.	Fringetree Bark
Chondrus crispus	Irish Moss
Cimicifuga racemosa Rad.	Black Cohosh Root
Cinnamomum zeylanicum Cort.	Cinammon Bark
Commiphora molmol	Myrrh Resin
Crataegus monogyna Flos.	Hawthorn Blossom
Crataegus monogyna Fruct.	Hawthorne Berry
Curcuma longa Rad.	Turmeric Tuber
Cynara scolymus Fol.	Artichoke Leaf
Dioscorea villosa Rad.	Wild Yam Root
Echinacea angustifolia Rad.	Coneflower Root
Eleutherococcus senticosus Rad.	Siberian Ginseng Root
Ephedra sinica Herba	Ma Huang Herb
Equisetum arvense Herba	Horsetail Herb
Erythraea centaurium Herba	Centaury Herb
Eschscholtzia californica Herba	Californian Poppy Herb

Alcohol & Tincturemaking Processes

Strength	% Alcohol	Suggested Process Type(s)
1:3, 1:1	45%	Infused, Macerated
1:3	45%	Decocted, Macerated
1:5, 1:3	25%, 45%	Decocted, Macerated
1:3	25%	Decocted, Macerated
1:3	25%	Decocted, Macerated
1:3	45%	Decocted, Macerated
1:3, 1:1	35%, 45%	Distilled, Decocted, Macerated
1:3	90%	Macerated
1:3, 1:1	25%, 45	Infused, Macerated
1:2, 1:1	25% 45%	Infused, Macerated
1:3, 1:1	70%	Macerated
1:3, 1:1	25%, 45%	Infused, Macerated
1:3	25%, 45%	Decocted, Macerated
1:3, 1:1	45%	Decocted, Macerated
1:3, 1:1	25%, 45%	Decocted, Macerated
1:3	25%, 45%	Macerated
1:3, 1:1	25%	Infused, Macerated
1:3	25%	Infused, Macerated
1:3, 1:1	45%	Infused, Macerated

The Formulary: Suggested Strength,

Latin Name	English Name
Eupatorium perfoliatum Herba	Boneset Herb
Eupatorium purpureum Rad.	Gravel Root
Euphrasia officinalis Herba	Eyebright Herb
Filipendula ulmaria Flos.	Meadowsweet Blossom
Foeniculum vulgare Sem.	Fennel Seed
Fucus vesiculosus Thallus	Bladderwrack
Fumaria offincinalis Herba	Fumitory Herb
Galega officinalis Herba	Goats Rue Herb
Galium aperine Herba	Cleavers Herb
Gelsemium sempervirens Rad	Yellow Jasmine Root
Gentiana lutea Rad.	Gentian Root
Geranium maculatum Rad.	American Cranesbill Root
Geum urbanum Rad.	Wood Avens Root
Ginkgo biloba Fol.	Ginkgo Leaf
Glechoma hederacea Herba	Ground Ivy Herb
Glycyrrhiza glabra Rad.	Liquorice Root
Grindelia robusta Herba.	Grindelia Herb
Guaiacum officinale Lig.	Guaiacum Wood
Gymnema sylvestre Fol.	Gurmar Leaf

Alcohol & Tincturemaking Processes

Strength	% Alcohol	Suggested Process Type(s)
1:3	25%, 45%	Infused, Macerated
1:3	25%, 45%	Decocted, Macerated
1:3, 1:1	25%, 45%	Infused, Macerated
1:3, 1:1	25%, 45%	Distilled, Infused, Macerated
1:3, 1:1	35%, 45%	Distilled, Infused, Macerated
1:3	25%	Macerated
1:3, 1:1	25%, 45%	Infused, Macerated
1:3	25%, 45%	Infused, Macerated
1:3, 1:1	25%	Infused, Macerated
1:10	60%	Macerated
1:3	45%	Decocted, Macerated
1:3	25%	Decocted, Macerated
1:3, 1:1	25%, 45%	Infused, Macerated
1:3, 1:1	25%, 45%	Infused, Macerated
1:3, 1:1	25%, 45%	Infused, Macerated
1:3, 1:1	25%	Decocted, Macerated
1:3	25%	Infused, Macerated
1:3	90%	Macerated
1:3	25%, 45%	Infused, Macerated

The Formulary: Suggested Strength,

Latin Name	English Name
Hamamelis virginiana Cort.	Witch Hazel Bark
Harpagophytum procumbens Rad.	Devils Claw Root
Humulus lupulus Flos.	Hops Strobiles
Hydrangea arborescens Rad.	Hydrangea Root
Hydrastis canadensis Rad.	Goldenseal Root
Hypericum perforatum Herba	St. John's Wort Herb
Hyssopus officinalis Herba	Hyssop Herb
Inula helenium Rad.	Elecampane Root
Iris versicolor Rad.	Blue Flag Rhizome
Junglans nigra Fol.	Black Walnut Leaf
Junglans nigra Fruct.	Black Walnut Hulls
Lactuca virosa Fol	Wild Lettuce Leaf
Lamium album Herba	White Dead Nettle Herb
Lavandula angustifolia Flos.	Lavender Flower
Leonurus cardiaca Herba	Motherwort Herb
Lobelia inflata Fol.	Lobelia Leaf
Lycium barbarum Fruct.	Goji Berry, Wolfberry
Lycopus virginicus Herba	Bugleweed Herb
Marrubium vulgare Herba.	White Horehound Herb

Alcohol & Tincturemaking Processes

Strength	% Alcohol	Suggested Process Type(s)
1:3	25%	Distilled, Decocted; Macerated
1:3, 1:1	25%	Decocted, Macerated
1:3, 1:1	60%	Macerated
1:3, 1:1	25%, 45%	Decocted, Macerated
1:3	60%	Decocted, Macerated
1:3, 1:1	60%	Infused, Macerated
1:3, 1:1	25%, 45%	Distilled, Infused, Macerated
1:3, 1:1	25%, 45%	Decocted, Macerated
1:3	25%, 45%	Decocted, Macerated
1:3	25%, 45%	Infused, Macerated
1:3	25%, 45%	Decocted, Macerated
1:3, 1:1	25%, 45%	Infused, Macerated
1:3, 1:1	25%, 45%	Infused, Macerated
1:3, 1:1	35%, 45%	Distilled, Infused, Macerated
1:3, 1:1	25%, 45%	Infused, Macerated
1:8	60%	Macerated
1:3, 1:1	25%	Decocted, Macerated
1:3, 1:1	25%, 45%	Infused, Macerated
1:3, 1:1	25%, 45%	Infused, Macerated

The Formulary: Suggested Strength,

Latin Name	English Name
Matricaria recutita Flos.	German Chamomile Flower
Medicago sativa Fol.	Alfalfa Tops
Melilotus officinalis Herba	Melilot Herb
Melissa officinalis Herba	Lemon Balm Herb
Mentha piperita Herba	Peppermint Herb
Mitchella repens Fruct.	Partridge Berry
Myrica cerifera Cort.	Bayberry Root Bark
Nepeta cataria Herba	Catnip Herb
Ocimum basilicum Herba	Basil Herb
Ocimum sanctum Herba	Tulsi Herb
Paeonia lactiflora Rad.	Paeony Root
Panax ginseng Rad.	Korean Ginseng Root
Parietaria diffusa Herba	Pellitory of the Wall Herb
Passiflora incarnata Flos.	Passion Flower
Peumus boldo Fol	Boldo Leaf
Phytolacca americana Rad.	Poke Root
Pimpinella anisum Sem.	Aniseed
Piscidia erythrina Cort.	Jamaican Dogwood Bark
Plantago lanceolata Fol.	Plantain Leaf

Alcohol & Tincturemaking Processes

Strength	% Alcohol	Suggested Process Type(s)
1:3, 1:1	45%	Distilled, Infused, Macerated
1:3, 1:1	25%	Infused, Macerated
1:3	25%, 45%	Infused, Macerated
1:3, 1:1	35%, 45%	Distilled then Macerated for 4 Hours.
1:3, 1:1	35%, 45%	Distilled, Infused, Macerated
1:3	25%, 45%	Infused; Macerated
1:3	35%, 45%	Decocted, Macerated
1:3, 1:1	25%, 45%	Infused, Macerated
1:2, 1:1	25%	Infused, Macerated
1:2, 1:1	25%	Infused, Macerated
1:3	25%, 45%	Decocted, Macerated
1:3	45%	Decocted, Macerated
1:3	25%	Infused, Macerated
1:3, 1:1	25%, 45%	Infused, Macerated
1:3	25%, 60%	Infused, Macerated
1:3	35%, 45%	Decocted, Macerated
1:3	35%, 45%	Distilled, Infused, Macerated
1:3	30%, 45%	Decocted, Macerated
1:2, 1:1	25%	Infused, Macerated

The Formulary: Suggested Strength,

Latin Name	English Name
Polygonatum odoratum Herba	Solomon's Seal Herb
Poria coccus	Tukahoe Fungus
Pulmonaria officinalis Herba	Lungwort Herb
Quercus robur Cort.	Oak Bark
Ranunculus ficaria Rad.	Lesser Celendine Root
Rheum officinale Rad.	Rhubarb Root
Rhodiola rosea Rad.	Gold Root
Rosa spp. Flos.	Rose Buds/Petals
Rosmarinus officinalis Herba	Rosemary Herb
Rubus idaeus Fol.	Raspberry Leaf
Rumex crispus Rad.	Yellow Dock Root
Salix alba Cort.	White Willow Bark
Salvia officinalis Herba	Sage Herb
Sambucus nigra Flos.	Elderflower
Sambucus nigra Fruct.	Elderberry
Schisandra chinensis Fruct.	Schisandra Berry
Scrophularia nodosa Herba	Figwort Herb
Scutellaria baicalensis Rad.	Baikal skullcap Root
Scutellaria lateriflora Herba.	Skullcap Herb

Alcohol & Tincturemaking Processes

Strength	% Alcohol	Suggested Process Type(s)
1:3	25%	Infused, Macerated
1:3, 1:1	25%	Decocted, Macerated
1:3	25%, 45%	Infused, Macerated
1:3	25%	Decocted, Macerated
1:5, 1:3	25%, 45%	Infused, Macerated
1:3	25%, 45%	Decocted, Macerated
1:3, 1:1	25%, 45%	Decocted, Macerated
1:3, 1:1	35%, 45%	Distilled, Infused, Macerated
1:3, 1:1	35%, 45%	Distilled, Infused, Macerated
1:3, 1:1	25%	Infused, Macerated
1:3, 1:1	25%, 45%	Decocted, Macerated
1:3, 1:1	25%, 45%	Decocted, Macerated
1:3, 1:1	25%, 45%	Distilled, Infused, Macerated
1:3, 1:1	25%	Infused, Macerated
1:2, 1:1	45%	Decocted, Macerated
1:3, 1:1	25%, 45%	Decocted, Macerated
1:3	25%, 45%	Infused, Macerated
1:3, 1:1	25%, 45%	Decocted, Macerated
1:3, 1:1	25%, 45%	Infused, Macerated

The Formulary: Suggested Strength,

Latin Name	English Name
Serenoa serrulata Fruct.	Saw Palmetto Berry
Smilax ornata Rad.	Sarsaparilla Root
Solidago virgaurea Fol.	Goldenrod Herb
Stachys betonica Herba	Wood Betony Herb
Stellaria media Herba	Chickweed Herb
Symphytum officinale Fol.	Comfrey Leaf
Symphytum officinale Rad.	Comfrey Root
Tabebuia impeteginosa Cort.	Pau D'Arco Bark
Tanacetum parthenium Herba	Feverfew Herb
Tanacetum vulgare Herba	Tansy Herb
Taraxacum officinale Fol.	Dandelion Leaf
Taraxacum officinale Rad.	Dandelion Root
Thuja occidentalis Fol.	Arbor Vitae Leaf
Thymus vulgaris Herba	Thyme Herb
Tilia europea Flos.	Limeflower
Trigonella foenum-grecum Sem.	Fenugreek Seed
Trifolium pratense Flos.	Red Clover Flowers
Trillium erectum Rad.	Beth Root
Turnera diffusa Fol.	Damiana Leaf

Alcohol & Tincturemaking Processes

Strength	% Alcohol	Suggested Process Type(s)
1:3, 1:1	75%	Macerated
1:3, 1:1	25%, 45%	Decocted, Macerated
1:3, 1:1	25%, 45%	Infused, Macerated
1:3, 1:1	25%, 45%	Infused, Macerated
1:3, 1:1	25%	Infused, Macerated
1:3, 1:1	25%	Macerated
1:3, 1:1	25%	Macerated
1:3, 1:1	45%	Decocted, Macerated
1:3, 1:1	25%, 45%	Infused, Macerated
1:3, 1:1	35%, 45%	Macerated
1:3, 1:1	25%, 45%	Infused, Macerated
1:3, 1:1	25%, 45%	Decocted, Macerated
1:10	60%	Distilled, Infused, Macerated
1:3, 1:1	45%	Distilled, Infused, Macerated
1:3, 1:1	25%	Infused, Macerated
1:3	25%, 45%	Decocted, Macerated
1:3, 1:1	25%, 45%	Infused, Macerated
1:3	45%	Macerated
1:3	45%, 60%	Distilled, Infused, Macerated

The Formulary: Suggested Strength,

Latin Name	English Name
Tussilago farfara Fol. & Flos.	Coltsfoot Flower/Leaf
Urtica dioica Fol.	Nettle Leaf/Herb
Urtica dioica Rad.	Nettle Root
Vaccinium myrtillus Fruct.	Bilberry
Valeriana officinalis Rad.	Valerian Root
Verbascum thapsus Fol.	Mullein Leaf
Verbena officinalis Herba	Vervain Herb
Viburnum opulus Cort.	Cramp Bark
Viburnum prunifolium Cort.	Black Haw Bark
Viola odorata Herba	Sweet Violet Herb
Viola tricolor Herba	Heartsease Herb
Viscum album Herba	Mistletoe Herb
Vitex agnus-castus Fruct.	Chaste Tree Berry
Withania somniferum Rad.	Ashwaganda Root
Zanthoxyllum americanum Cort.	Prickly Ash Bark
Zea mays Stigmata	Cornsilk
Zingiber officinale Rad.	Ginger Tuber

Alcohol & Tincturemaking Processes

Strength	% Alcohol	Suggested Process Type(s)
1:3, 1:1	25%, 45%	Infused, Macerated
1:3, 1:1	25%, 45%	Infused, Macerated
1:3, 1:1	25%, 45%	Decocted, Macerated
1:3, 1:1	25%	Decocted, Macerated
1:3, 1:1	25%, 45%	Decocted, Macerated
1:3, 1:1	25%, 45%	Infused, Macerated
1:3, 1:1	25%, 45%	Infused, Macerated
1:3, 1:1	25%, 45%	Decocted, Macerated
1:3, 1:1	25%	Decocted, Macerated
1:3	25%	Infused, Macerated
1:3	25%, 45%	Infused, Macerated
1:3, 1:1	25%, 45%	Macerated
1:3, 1:1	25%, 45%	Distilled, Decocted, Macerated
1:3, 1:1	45%	Decocted, Macerated
1:3, 1:1	45%	Decocted, Macerated
1:3, 1:1	25%, 45%	Infused, Macerated
1:2, 1:1	90%	Distilled, Infused, Macerated

Part 3

The Cheat-Sheets:

Lookup tables of amounts

1:5   25%   (Vodka)   Dried Herb

Dried Herb	Vodka 37.5%	Added water	Total Menstruum
10 g	33 ml	17 ml	50 ml
20 g	66 ml	33 ml	100 ml
25 g	83 ml	42 ml	125 ml
30 g	100 ml	50 ml	150 ml
50 g	166 ml	83 ml	250 ml
75 g	250 ml	125 ml	375 ml
100 g	333 ml	167 ml	500 ml
125 g	416 ml	208 ml	625 ml
150 g	500 ml	250 ml	750 ml
200 g	666 ml	333 ml	1000 ml
250 g	833 ml	417 ml	1.25 L

1:4   25%   (Vodka)   Dried Herb

Dried Herb	Vodka 37.5%	Added water	Total Menstruum
10 g	26 ml	13 ml	40 ml
20 g	53 ml	27 ml	80 ml
25 g	66 ml	33 ml	100 ml
30 g	80 ml	40 ml	120 ml
50 g	133 ml	67 ml	200 ml
75 g	200 ml	100 ml	300 ml
100 g	266 ml	133 ml	400 ml
125 g	333 ml	167 ml	500 ml
150 g	400 ml	200 ml	600 ml
200 g	533 ml	267 ml	800 ml
250 g	666 ml	333 ml	1000 ml

1:3   25%   (Vodka)   Dried Herb

Dried Herb	Vodka 37.5%	Added water	Total Menstruum
10 g	20ml	10 ml	30 ml
20 g	40 ml	20 ml	60 ml
25 g	50 ml	25 ml	75 ml
30 g	60 ml	30 ml	90 ml
50 g	100 ml	50 ml	150 ml
75 g	150 ml	75 ml	225 ml
100 g	200 ml	100 ml	300 ml
125 g	250 ml	125 ml	375 ml
150 g	300 ml	150 ml	450 ml
200 g	400 ml	200 ml	600 ml
250 g	500 ml	250 ml	750 ml

1:5   35%   (Vodka)   Dried Herb

Dried Herb	Vodka 37.5%	Added water	Total Menstruum
10 g	46 ml	3 ml	50 ml
20 g	93 ml	7 ml	100 ml
25 g	116 ml	8 ml	125 ml
30 g	140 ml	10 ml	150 ml
50 g	233 ml	17 ml	250 ml
75 g	350 ml	25 ml	375 ml
100 g	466 ml	33 ml	500 ml
125 g	583 ml	42 ml	625 ml
150 g	700 ml	50 ml	750 ml
200 g	933 ml	67 ml	1.00 L
250 g	1.16 L	83 ml	1.25 L

1:4   35%   (Vodka)   Dried Herb

Dried Herb	Vodka 37.5%	Added water	Total Menstruum
10 g	37 ml	3 ml	40 ml
20 g	74 ml	5 ml	80 ml
25 g	93 ml	7 ml	100 ml
30 g	112 ml	8 ml	120 ml
50 g	186 ml	13 ml	200 ml
75 g	280 ml	20 ml	300 ml
100 g	373 ml	27 ml	400 ml
125 g	466 ml	33 ml	500 ml
150 g	560 ml	40 ml	600 ml
200 g	746 ml	53 ml	800 ml
250 g	933 ml	67 ml	1.00 L

1:3 35% (Vodka) Dried Herb

Dried Herb	Vodka 37.5%	Added water	Total Menstruum
10 g	28 ml	2 ml	30 ml
20 g	56 ml	4 ml	60 ml
25 g	70 ml	5 ml	75 ml
30 g	84 ml	6 ml	90 ml
50 g	140 ml	10 ml	150 ml
75 g	210 ml	15 ml	225 ml
100 g	280 ml	20 ml	300 ml
125 g	350 ml	25 ml	375 ml
150 g	420 ml	30 ml	450 ml
200 g	560 ml	40 ml	600 ml
250 g	700 ml	50 ml	750 ml

1:5   25%   (Vodka)   Fresh Herb

Fresh Herb	Vodka 37.5%	Added water	Total Menstruum
10 g	33 ml	9 ml	50 ml
20 g	66 ml	18 ml	100 ml
25 g	83 ml	23 ml	125 ml
30 g	100 ml	28 ml	150 ml
50 g	166 ml	46 ml	250 ml
75 g	250 ml	69 ml	375 ml
100 g	333 ml	92 ml	500 ml
125 g	416 ml	115 ml	625 ml
150 g	500 ml	138 ml	750 ml
200 g	666 ml	183 ml	1.00 L
250 g	833 ml	229 ml	1.25 L

This formula assumes the fresh herb contains 75% water by weight

1:4   25%   (Vodka)   Fresh Herb

Fresh Herb	Vodka 37.5%	Added water	Total Menstruum
10 g	26 ml	6 ml	40 ml
20 g	53 ml	12 ml	80 ml
25 g	66 ml	15 ml	100 ml
30 g	80 ml	18 ml	120 ml
50 g	133 ml	29 ml	200 ml
75 g	200 ml	44 ml	300 ml
100 g	266 ml	58 ml	400 ml
125 g	333 ml	73 ml	500 ml
150 g	400 ml	88 ml	600 ml
200 g	533 ml	117 ml	800 ml
250 g	666 ml	146 ml	1.00 L

This formula assumes the fresh herb contains 75% water by weight

1:3   25%   (Vodka)   Fresh Herb

Fresh Herb	Vodka 37.5%	Added water	Total Menstruum
10 g	20 ml	3 ml	30 ml
20 g	40 ml	5 ml	60 ml
25 g	50 ml	6 ml	75 ml
30 g	60 ml	7 ml	90 ml
50 g	100 ml	13 ml	150 ml
75 g	150 ml	19 ml	225 ml
100 g	200 ml	25 ml	300 ml
125 g	250 ml	31 ml	375 ml
150 g	300 ml	38 ml	450 ml
200 g	400 ml	50 ml	600 ml
250 g	500 ml	63 ml	750 ml

This formula assumes the fresh herb contains 75% water by weight

1:10   25% (Ethanol)   Dried Herb

Dried Herb	Ethanol	Added water	Total Menstruum
50 g	125 ml	375 ml	500 ml
100 g	250 ml	750 ml	1.00 L
150 g	375 ml	1.12 L	1.50 L
200 g	500 ml	1.50 L	2.00 L
250 g	625 ml	1.87 L	2.50 L
300 g	750 ml	2.25 L	3.00 L
400 g	1.00 L	3.00 L	4.00 L
500 g	1.25 L	3.75 L	5.00 L
600 g	1.50 L	4.50 L	6.00 L
700 g	1.75 L	5.25 L	7.00 L
800 g	2.00 L	6.00 L	8.00 L
900 g	2.25 L	6.75 L	9.00 L
1.00 Kg	2.50 L	7.50 L	10.00 L
1.25 Kg	3.13 L	9.38 L	12.50 L
1.50 Kg	3.75 L	11.25 L	15.00 L
1.75 Kg	4.38 L	13.13 L	17.50 L
2.00 Kg	5.00 L	15.00 L	20.00 L
2.50 Kg	6.25 L	18.75 L	25.00 L
3.00 Kg	7.50 L	22.50 L	30.00 L

1:8 25% (Ethanol)   Dried Herb

Dried Herb	Ethanol	Added water	Total Menstruum
50 g	100 ml	300 ml	400 ml
100 g	200 ml	600 ml	800 ml
150 g	300 ml	900 ml	1.20 L
200 g	400 ml	1.20 L	1.60 L
250 g	500 ml	1.50 L	2.00 L
300 g	600 ml	1.80 L	2.40 L
400 g	800 ml	2.40 L	3.20 L
500 g	1.00 L	3.00 L	4.00 L
600 g	1.20 L	3.60 L	4.80 L
700 g	1.40 L	4.20 L	5.60 L
800 g	1.60 L	4.80 L	6.40 L
900 g	1.80 L	5.40 L	7.20 L
1.00 Kg	2.00 L	6.00 L	8.00 L
1.25 Kg	2.50 L	7.50 L	10.00 L
1.50 Kg	3.00 L	9.00 L	12.00 L
1.75 Kg	3.50 L	10.50 L	14.00 L
2.00 Kg	4.00 L	12.00 L	16.00 L
2.50 Kg	5.00 L	15.00 L	20.00 L
3.00 Kg	6.00 L	18.00 L	24.00 L

1:6 25% (Ethanol) Dried Herb

Dried Herb	Ethanol	Added water	Total Menstruum
50 g	75 ml	225 ml	300 ml
100 g	150 ml	450 ml	600 ml
150 g	225 ml	675 ml	900 ml
200 g	300 ml	900 ml	1.20 L
250 g	375 ml	1.12 L	1.50 L
300 g	450 ml	1.35 L	1.80 L
400 g	600 ml	1.80 L	2.40 L
500 g	750 ml	2.25 L	3.00 L
600 g	900 ml	2.70 L	3.60 L
700 g	1.05 L	3.15 L	4.20 L
800 g	1.20 L	3.60 L	4.80 L
900 g	1.35 L	4.05 L	5.40 L
1.00 Kg	1.50 L	4.50 L	6.00 L
1.25 Kg	1.88 L	5.63 L	7.50 L
1.50 Kg	2.25 L	6.75 L	9.00 L
1.75 Kg	2.63 L	7.88 L	10.50 L
2.00 Kg	3.00 L	9.00 L	12.00 L
2.50 Kg	3.75 L	11.25 L	15.00 L
3.00 Kg	4.50 L	13.50 L	18.00 L

1:5   25% (Ethanol)   Dried Herb

Dried Herb	Ethanol	Added water	Total Menstruum
50 g	62 ml	188 ml	250 ml
100 g	125 ml	375 ml	500 ml
150 g	187 ml	563 ml	750 ml
200 g	250 ml	750 ml	1 L
250 g	312 ml	938 ml	1.25 L
300 g	375 ml	1.12 L	1.5 L
400 g	500 ml	1.5 L	2 L
500 g	625 ml	1.87 L	2.5 L
600 g	750 ml	2.25 L	3 Ll
700 g	875 ml	2.62 L	3.50 L
800 g	1 L	3 L	4.00 L
900 g	1.12 L	3.37 L	4.50 L
1.00 Kg	1.25 L	3.75 L	5.00 L
1.25 Kg	1.56 L	4.69 L	6.25 L
1.50 Kg	1.88 L	5.63 L	7.50 L
1.75 Kg	2.19 L	6.56 L	8.75 L
2.00 Kg	2.50 L	7.50 L	10.00 L
2.50 Kg	3.13 L	9.38 L	12.50 L
3.00 Kg	3.75 L	11.25 L	15.00 L

1:4 25% (Ethanol)   Dried Herb

Dried Herb	Ethanol	Added water	Total Menstruum
50 g	50 ml	150 ml	200 ml
100 g	100 ml	300 ml	400 ml
150 g	150 ml	450 ml	600 ml
200 g	200 ml	600 ml	800 ml
250 g	250 ml	750 ml	1.00 L
300 g	300 ml	900 ml	1.20 L
400 g	400 ml	1.20 L	1.60 L
500 g	500 ml	1.50 L	2.00 L
600 g	600 ml	1.80 L	2.40 L
700 g	700 ml	2.10 L	2.80 L
800 g	800 ml	2.40 L	3.20 L
900 g	900 ml	2.70 L	3.60 L
1.00 Kg	1.00 L	3.00 L	4.00 L
1.25 Kg	1.25 L	3.75 L	5.00 L
1.50 Kg	1.50 L	4.50 L	6.00 L
1.75 Kg	1.75 L	5.25 L	7.00 L
2.00 Kg	2.00 L	6.00 L	8.00 L
2.50 Kg	2.50 L	7.50 L	10.00 L
3.00 Kg	3.00 L	9.00 L	12.00 L

1:3   25%   (Ethanol)   Dried Herb

Dried Herb	Ethanol	Added water	Total Menstruum
50 g	37 ml	113 ml	150 ml
100 g	75 ml	225 ml	300 ml
150 g	112 ml	338 ml	450 ml
200 g	150 ml	450 ml	600 ml
250 g	187 ml	563 ml	750 ml
300 g	225 ml	675 ml	900 ml
400 g	300 ml	900 ml	1.20 L
500 g	375 ml	1.12 L	1.50 L
600 g	450 ml	1.35 L	1.80 L
700 g	525 ml	1.57 L	2.10 L
800 g	600 ml	1.80 L	2.40 L
900 g	675 ml	2.02 L	2.70 L
1.00 Kg	750 ml	2.25 L	3.00 L
1.25 Kg	940 ml	2.81 L	3.75 L
1.50 Kg	1.13 L	3.38 L	4.50 L
1.75 Kg	1.31 L	3.94 L	5.25 L
2.00 Kg	1.50 L	4.50 L	6.00 L
2.50 Kg	1.88 L	5.63 L	7.50 L
3.00 Kg	2.25 L	6.75 L	9.00 L

1:2   25% (Ethanol)   Dried Herb

Dried Herb	Ethanol	Added water	Total Menstruum
50 g	25 ml	75 ml	100 ml
100 g	50 ml	150 ml	200 ml
150 g	75 ml	225 ml	300 ml
200 g	100 ml	300 ml	400 ml
250 g	125 ml	375 ml	500 ml
300 g	150 ml	450 ml	600 ml
400 g	200 ml	600 ml	800 ml
500 g	250 ml	750 ml	1.00 L
600 g	300 ml	900 ml	1.20 L
700 g	350 ml	1.05 L	1.40 L
800 g	400 ml	1.20 L	1.60 L
900 g	450 ml	1.35 L	1.80 L
1.00 Kg	500 ml	1.50 L	2.00 L
1.25 Kg	620 ml	1.88 L	2.50 L
1.50 Kg	750 ml	2.25 L	3.00 L
1.75 Kg	880 ml	2.62 L	3.50 L
2.00 Kg	1.00 L	3.00 L	4.00 L
2.50 Kg	1.25 L	3.75 L	5.00 L
3.00 Kg	1.50 L	4.50 L	6.00 L

1:1   25% (Ethanol)   F.E.   Dried Herb

Dried Herb	Ethanol	Added water	Total Menstruum
50 g	12 ml	38 ml	50 ml
100 g	25 ml	75 ml	100 ml
150 g	37 ml	113 ml	150 ml
200 g	50 ml	150 ml	200 ml
250 g	62 ml	188 ml	250 ml
300 g	75 ml	225 ml	300 ml
400 g	100 ml	300 ml	400 ml
500 g	125 ml	375 ml	500 ml
600 g	150 ml	450 ml	600 ml
700 g	175 ml	525 ml	700 ml
800 g	200 ml	600 ml	800 ml
900 g	225 ml	675 ml	900 ml
1.00 Kg	250 ml	750 ml	1.00 L
1.25 Kg	310 ml	940 ml	1.25 L
1.50 Kg	380 ml	1.13 L	1.50 L
1.75 Kg	440 ml	1.31 L	1.75 L
2.00 Kg	500 ml	1.50 L	2.00 L
2.50 Kg	630 ml	1.88 L	2.50 L
3.00 Kg	750 ml	2.25 L	3.00 L

1:5 35% (Ethanol)   Dried Herb

Dried Herb	Ethanol	Added water	Total Menstruum
50 g	87 ml	163 ml	250 ml
100 g	175 ml	325 ml	500 ml
150 g	262 ml	488 ml	750 ml
200 g	350 ml	650 ml	1.00 L
250 g	437 ml	813 ml	1.25 L
300 g	525 ml	975 ml	1.50 L
400 g	700 ml	1.30 L	2.00 L
500 g	875 ml	1.62 L	2.50 L
600 g	1.05 L	1.95 L	3.00 L
700 g	1.22 L	2.27 L	3.50 L
800 g	1.40 L	2.60 L	4.00 L
900 g	1.57 L	2.92 L	4.50 L
1.00 Kg	1.75 L	3.25 L	5.00 L
1.25 Kg	2.19 L	4.06 L	6.25 L
1.50 Kg	2.63 L	4.88 L	7.50 L
1.75 Kg	3.06 L	5.69 L	8.75 L
2.00 Kg	3.50 L	6.50 L	10.00 L
2.50 Kg	4.38 L	8.13 L	12.50 L
3.00 Kg	5.25 L	9.75 L	15.00 L

1:4 35% (Ethanol)   Dried Herb

Dried Herb	Ethanol	Added water	Total Menstruum
50 g	70 ml	130 ml	200 ml
100 g	140 ml	260 ml	400 ml
150 g	210 ml	390 ml	600 ml
200 g	280 ml	520 ml	800 ml
250 g	350 ml	650 ml	1.00 L
300 g	420 ml	780 ml	1.20 L
400 g	560 ml	1.04 L	1.60 L
500 g	700 ml	1.30 L	2.00 L
600 g	840 ml	1.56 L	2.40 L
700 g	980 ml	1.82 L	2.80 L
800 g	1.12 L	2.08 L	3.20 L
900 g	1.26 L	2.34 L	3.60 L
1.00 Kg	1.40 L	2.60 L	4.00 L
1.25 Kg	1.75 L	3.25 L	5.00 L
1.50 Kg	2.10 L	3.90 L	6.00 L
1.75 Kg	2.45 L	4.55 L	7.00 L
2.00 Kg	2.80 L	5.20 L	8.00 L
2.50 Kg	3.50 L	6.50 L	10.00 L
3.00 Kg	4.20 L	7.80 L	12.00 L

1:3 35% (Ethanol)   Dried Herb

Dried Herb	Ethanol	Added water	Total Menstruum
50 g	52 ml	98 ml	150 ml
100 g	105 ml	195 ml	300 ml
150 g	157 ml	293 ml	450 ml
200 g	210 ml	390 ml	600 ml
250 g	262 ml	488 ml	750 ml
300 g	315 ml	585 ml	900 ml
400 g	420 ml	780 ml	1.20 L
500 g	525 ml	975 ml	1.50 L
600 g	630 ml	1.17 L	1.80 L
700 g	735 ml	1.36 L	2.10 L
800 g	840 ml	1.56 L	2.40 L
900 g	945 ml	1.75 L	2.70 L
1.00 Kg	1.05 L	1.95 L	3.00 L
1.25 Kg	1.31 L	2.44 L	3.75 L
1.50 Kg	1.58 L	2.93 L	4.50 L
1.75 Kg	1.84 L	3.41 L	5.25 L
2.00 Kg	2.10 L	3.90 L	6.00 L
2.50 Kg	2.63 L	4.88 L	7.50 L
3.00 Kg	3.15 L	5.85 L	9.00 L

1:2 35% (Ethanol) Dried Herb

Dried Herb	Ethanol	Added water	Total Menstruum
50 g	35 ml	65 ml	100 ml
100 g	70 ml	130 ml	200 ml
150 g	105 ml	195 ml	300 ml
200 g	140 ml	260 ml	400 ml
250 g	175 ml	325 ml	500 ml
300 g	210 ml	390 ml	600 ml
400 g	280 ml	520 ml	800 ml
500 g	350 ml	650 ml	1.00 L
600 g	420 ml	780 ml	1.20 L
700 g	490 ml	910 ml	1.40 L
800 g	560 ml	1.04 L	1.60 L
900 g	630 ml	1.17 L	1.80 L
1.00 Kg	700 ml	1.30 L	2.00 L
1.25 Kg	880 ml	1.63 L	2.50 L
1.50 Kg	1.05 L	1.95 L	3.00 L
1.75 Kg	1.23 L	2.28 L	3.50 L
2.00 Kg	1.40 L	2.60 L	4.00 L
2.50 Kg	1.75 L	3.25 L	5.00 L
3.00 Kg	2.10 L	3.90 L	6.00 L

1:1 35% (Ethanol) F.E.   Dried Herb

Dried Herb	Ethanol	Added water	Total Menstruum
50 g	17 ml	33 ml	50 ml
100 g	35 ml	65 ml	100 ml
150 g	52 ml	98 ml	150 ml
200 g	70 ml	130 ml	200 ml
250 g	87 ml	163 ml	250 ml
300 g	105 ml	195 ml	300 ml
400 g	140 ml	260 ml	400 ml
500 g	175 ml	325 ml	500 ml
600 g	210 ml	390 ml	600 ml
700 g	245 ml	455 ml	700 ml
800 g	280 ml	520 ml	800 ml
900 g	315 ml	585 ml	900 ml
1.00 Kg	350 ml	650 ml	1.00 L
1.25 Kg	440 ml	810 ml	1.25 L
1.50 Kg	530 ml	980 ml	1.50 L
1.75 Kg	610 ml	1.14 L	1.75 L
2.00 Kg	700 ml	1.30 L	2.00 L
2.50 Kg	880 ml	1.63 L	2.50 L
3.00 Kg	1.05 L	1.95 L	3.00 L

1:10 45% (Ethanol) Dried Herb

Dried Herb	Ethanol	Added water	Total Menstruum
50 g	225 ml	275 ml	500 ml
100 g	450 ml	550 ml	1.00 L
150 g	675 ml	825 ml	1.50 L
200 g	900 ml	1.10 L	2.00 L
250 g	1.12 L	1.37 L	2.50 L
300 g	1.35 L	1.65 L	3.00 L
400 g	1.80 L	2.20 L	4.00 L
500 g	2.25 L	2.75 L	5.00 L
600 g	2.70 L	3.30 L	6.00 L
700 g	3.15 L	3.85 L	7.00 L
800 g	3.60 L	4.40 L	8.00 L
900 g	4.05 L	4.95 L	9.00 L
1.00 Kg	4.50 L	5.50 L	10.00 L
1.25 Kg	5.63 L	6.88 L	12.50 L
1.50 Kg	6.75 L	8.25 L	15.00 L
1.75 Kg	7.88 L	9.63 L	17.50 L
2.00 Kg	9.00 L	11.00 L	20.00 L
2.50 Kg	11.25 L	13.75 L	25.00 L
3.00 Kg	13.50 L	16.50 L	30.00 L

1:8 45% (Ethanol)   Dried Herb

Dried Herb	Ethanol	Added water	Total Menstruum
50 g	180 ml	220 ml	400 ml
100 g	360 ml	440 ml	800 ml
150 g	540 ml	660 ml	1.20 L
200 g	720 ml	880 ml	1.60 L
250 g	900 ml	1.10 L	2.00 L
300 g	1.08 L	1.32 L	2.40 L
400 g	1.44 L	1.76 L	3.20 L
500 g	1.80 L	2.20 L	4.00 L
600 g	2.16 L	2.64 L	4.80 L
700 g	2.52 L	3.08 L	5.60 L
800 g	2.88 L	3.52 L	6.40 L
900 g	3.24 L	3.96 L	7.20 L
1.00 Kg	3.60 L	4.40 L	8.00 L
1.25 Kg	4.50 L	5.50 L	10.00 L
1.50 Kg	5.40 L	6.60 L	12.00 L
1.75 Kg	6.30 L	7.70 L	14.00 L
2.00 Kg	7.20 L	8.80 L	16.00 L
2.50 Kg	9.00 L	11.00 L	20.00 L
3.00 Kg	10.80 L	13.20 L	24.00 L

1:5   45% (Ethanol)   Dried Herb

Dried Herb	Ethanol	Added water	Total Menstruum
50 g	112 ml	138 ml	250 ml
100 g	225 ml	275 ml	500 ml
150 g	337 ml	413 ml	750 ml
200 g	450 ml	550 ml	1.00 L
250 g	562 ml	688 ml	1.25 L
300 g	675 ml	825 ml	1.50 L
400 g	900 ml	1.10 L	2.00 L
500 g	1.12 L	1.37 L	2.50 L
600 g	1.35 L	1.65 L	3.00 L
700 g	1.57 L	1.92 L	3.50 L
800 g	1.80 L	2.20 L	4.00 L
900 g	2.02 L	2.47 L	4,50 L
1.00 Kg	2.25 L	2.75 L	5.00 L
1.25 Kg	2.81 L	3.44 L	6.25 L
1.50 Kg	3.38 L	4.13 L	7.50 L
1.75 Kg	3.94 L	4.81 L	8.75 L
2.00 Kg	4.50 L	5.50 L	10.00 L
2.50 Kg	5.63 L	6.88 L	12.50 L
3.00 Kg	6.75 L	8.25 L	15.00 L

1:4   45% (Ethanol)   Dried Herb

Dried Herb	Ethanol	Added water	Total Menstruum
50 g	90 ml	110 ml	200 ml
100 g	180 ml	220 ml	400 ml
150 g	270 ml	330 ml	600 ml
200 g	360 ml	440 ml	800 ml
250 g	450 ml	550 ml	1.00 L
300 g	540 ml	660 ml	1.20 L
400 g	720 ml	880 ml	1.60 L
500 g	900 ml	1.10 L	2.00 L
600 g	1.08 L	1.32 L	2.40 L
700 g	1.26 L	1.54 L	2.80 L
800 g	1.44 L	1.76 L	3.20 L
900 g	1.62 L	1.98 L	3.60 L
1.00 Kg	1.80 L	2.20 L	4.00 L
1.25 Kg	2.25 L	2.75 L	5.00 L
1.50 Kg	2.70 L	3.30 L	6.00 L
1.75 Kg	3.15 L	3.85 L	7.00 L
2.00 Kg	3.60 L	4.40 L	8.00 L
2.50 Kg	4.50 L	5.50 L	10.00 L
3.00 Kg	5.40 L	6.60 L	12.00 L

1:3   45% (Ethanol)   Dried Herb

Dried Herb	Ethanol	Added water	Total Menstruum
50 g	67 ml	83 ml	150 ml
100 g	135 ml	165 ml	300 ml
150 g	202 ml	248 ml	450 ml
200 g	270 ml	330 ml	600 ml
250 g	337 ml	413 ml	750 ml
300 g	405 ml	495 ml	900 ml
400 g	540 ml	660 ml	1.20 L
500 g	675 ml	825 ml	1.50 L
600 g	810 ml	990 ml	1.80 L
700 g	945 ml	1.15 L	2.10 L
800 g	1.08 L	1.32 L	2.40 L
900 g	1.21 L	1.48 L	2.70 L
1.00 Kg	1.35 L	1.65 L	3.00 L
1.25 Kg	1.69 L	2.06 L	3.75 L
1.50 Kg	2.03 L	2.48 L	4.50 L
1.75 Kg	2.36 L	2.89 L	5.25 L
2.00 Kg	2.70 L	3.30 L	6.00 L
2.50 Kg	3.38 L	4.13 L	7.50 L
3.00 Kg	4.05 L	4.95 L	9.00 L

1:2 45% (Ethanol)   Dried Herb

Dried Herb	Ethanol	Added water	Total Menstruum
50 g	45 ml	55 ml	100 ml
100 g	90 ml	110 ml	200 ml
150 g	135 ml	165 ml	300 ml
200 g	180 ml	220 ml	400 ml
250 g	225 ml	275 ml	500 ml
300 g	270 ml	330 ml	600 ml
400 g	360 ml	440 ml	800 ml
500 g	450 ml	550 ml	1.00 L
600 g	540 ml	660 ml	1.20 L
700 g	630 ml	770 ml	1.40 L
800 g	720 ml	880 ml	1.60 L
900 g	810 ml	990 ml	1.80 L
1.00 Kg	900 ml	1.10 L	2.00 L
1.25 Kg	1.13 L	1.38 L	2.50 L
1.50 Kg	1.35 L	1.65 L	3.00 L
1.75 Kg	1.58 L	1.93 L	3.50 L
2.00 Kg	1.80 L	2.20 L	4.00 L
2.50 Kg	2.25 L	2.75 L	5.00 L
3.00 Kg	2.70 L	3.30 L	6.00 L

1:1 45% (Ethanol) F.E.   Dried Herb

Dried Herb	Ethanol	Added water	Total Menstruum
50 g	22 ml	28 ml	50 ml
100 g	45 ml	55 ml	100 ml
150 g	67 ml	83 ml	150 ml
200 g	90 ml	110 ml	200 ml
250 g	112 ml	138 ml	250 ml
300 g	135 ml	165 ml	300 ml
400 g	180 ml	220 ml	400 ml
500 g	225 ml	275 ml	500 ml
600 g	270 ml	330 ml	600 ml
700 g	315 ml	385 ml	700 ml
800 g	360 ml	440 ml	800 ml
900 g	405 ml	495 ml	900 ml
1.00 Kg	450 ml	550 ml	1.00 L
1.25 Kg	650 ml	690 ml	1.25 L
1.50 Kg	680 ml	830 ml	1.50 L
1.75 Kg	790 ml	960 ml	1.75 L
2.00 Kg	900 ml	1.10 L	2.00 L
2.50 Kg	1.13 L	1.38 L	2.50 L
3.00 Kg	1.35 L	1.65 L	3.00 L

1:5   60% (Ethanol)   Dried Herb

Dried Herb	Ethanol	Added water	Total Menstruum
50 g	150 ml	100 ml	250 ml
100 g	300 ml	200 ml	500 ml
150 g	450 ml	300 ml	750 ml
200 g	600 ml	400 ml	1.00 L
250 g	750 ml	500 ml	1.25 L
300 g	900 ml	600 ml	1.50 L
400 g	1.20 L	800 ml	2.00 L
500 g	1.50 L	1.00 L	2.50 L
600 g	1.80 L	1.20 L	3.00 L
700 g	2.10 L	1.40 L	3.50 L
800 g	2.40 L	1.60 L	4.00 L
900 g	2.70 L	1.80 L	4.50 L
1.00 Kg	3.00 L	2.00 L	5.00 L
1.25 Kg	3.75 L	2.50 L	6.25 L
1.50 Kg	4.50 L	3.00 L	7.50 L
1.75 Kg	5.25 L	3.50 L	8.75 L
2.00 Kg	6.00 L	4.00 L	10.00 L
2.50 Kg	7.50 L	5.00 L	12.50 L
3.00 Kg	9.00 L	6.00 L	15.00 L

1:4 60% (Ethanol)   Dried Herb

Dried Herb	Ethanol	Added water	Total Menstruum
50 g	120 ml	80 ml	200 ml
100 g	240 ml	160 ml	400 ml
150 g	360 ml	240 ml	600 ml
200 g	480 ml	320 ml	800 ml
250 g	600 ml	400 ml	1.00 L
300 g	720 ml	480 ml	1.20 L
400 g	960 ml	640 ml	1.60 L
500 g	1.20 L	800 ml	2.00 L
600 g	1.44 L	960 ml	2.40 L
700 g	1.68 L	1.12 L	2.80 L
800 g	1.92 L	1.28 L	3.20 L
900 g	2.16 L	1.44 L	3.60 L
1.00 Kg	2.40 L	1.60 L	4.00 L
1.25 Kg	3.00 L	2.00 L	5.00 L
1.50 Kg	3.60 L	2.40 L	6.00 L
1.75 Kg	4.20 L	2.80 L	7.00 L
2.00 Kg	4.80 L	3.20 L	8.00 L
2.50 Kg	6.00 L	4.00 L	10.00 L
3.00 Kg	7.20 L	4.80 L	12.00 L

1:3   60% (Ethanol)   Dried Herb

Dried Herb	Ethanol	Added water	Total Menstruum
50 g	90 ml	60 ml	150 ml
100 g	180 ml	120 ml	300 ml
150 g	270 ml	180 ml	450 ml
200 g	360 ml	240 ml	600 ml
250 g	450 ml	300 ml	750 ml
300 g	540 ml	360 ml	900 ml
400 g	720 ml	480 ml	1.20 L
500 g	900 ml	600 ml	1.50 L
600 g	1.08 L	720 ml	1.80 L
700 g	1.26 L	840 ml	2.10 L
800 g	1.44 L	960 ml	2.40 L
900 g	1.62 L	1.08 L	2.70 L
1.00 Kg	1.80 L	1.20 L	3.00 L
1.25 Kg	2.25 L	1.50 L	3.75 L
1.50 Kg	2.70 L	1.80 L	4.50 L
1.75 Kg	3.15 L	2.10 L	5.25 L
2.00 Kg	3.60 L	2.40 L	6.00 L
2.50 Kg	4.50 L	3.00 L	7.50 L
3.00 Kg	5.40 L	3.60 L	9.00 L

1:2 60% (Ethanol)   Dried Herb

Dried Herb	Ethanol	Added water	Total Menstruum
50 g	60 ml	40 ml	100 ml
100 g	120 ml	80 ml	200 ml
150 g	180 ml	120 ml	300 ml
200 g	240 ml	160 ml	400 ml
250 g	300 ml	200 ml	500 ml
300 g	360 ml	240 ml	600 ml
400 g	480 ml	320 ml	800 ml
500 g	600 ml	400 ml	1.00 L
600 g	720 ml	480 ml	1.20 L
700 g	840 ml	560 ml	1.40 L
800 g	960 ml	640 ml	1.60 L
900 g	1.08 L	720 ml	1.80 L
1.00 Kg	1.20 L	800 ml	2.00 L
1.25 Kg	1.50 L	1.00 L	2.50 L
1.50 Kg	1.80 L	1.20 L	3.00 L
1.75 Kg	2.10 L	1.40 L	3.50 L
2.00 Kg	2.40 L	1.60 L	4.00 L
2.50 Kg	3.00 L	2.00 L	5.00 L
3.00 Kg	3.60 L	2.40 L	6.00 L

1:1   60% (Ethanol) F.E.   Dried Herb

Dried Herb	Ethanol	Added water	Total Menstruum
50 g	30 ml	20 ml	50 ml
100 g	60 ml	40 ml	100 ml
150 g	90 ml	60 ml	150 ml
200 g	120 ml	80 ml	200 ml
250 g	150 ml	100 ml	250 ml
300 g	180 ml	120 ml	300 ml
400 g	240 ml	160 ml	400 ml
500 g	300 ml	200 ml	500 ml
600 g	360 ml	240 ml	600 ml
700 g	420 ml	280 ml	700 ml
800 g	480 ml	320 ml	800 ml
900 g	540 ml	360 ml	900 ml
1.00 Kg	600 ml	400 ml	1.00 L
1.25 Kg	750 ml	500 ml	1.25 L
1.50 Kg	900 ml	600 ml	1.50 L
1.75 Kg	1.05 L	700 ml	1.75 L
2.00 Kg	1.20 L	800 ml	2.00 L
2.50 Kg	1.50 L	1.00 L	2.50 L
3.00 Kg	1.80 L	1.20 L	3.00 L

1:5   90% (Ethanol)   Dried Herb

Dried Herb	Ethanol	Added water	Total Menstruum
50 g	225 ml	25 ml	250 ml
100 g	450 ml	50 ml	500 ml
150 g	675 ml	75 ml	750 ml
200 g	900 ml	100 ml	1.00 L
250 g	1.12 L	125 ml	1.25 L
300 g	1.35 L	150 ml	1.50 L
400 g	1.80 L	200 ml	2.00 L
500 g	2.25 L	250 ml	2.50 L
600 g	2.70 L	300 ml	3.00 L
700 g	3.15 L	350 ml	3.50 L
800 g	3.60 L	400 ml	4.00 L
900 g	4.05 L	450 ml	4.50 L
1.00 Kg	4.50 L	500 ml	5.00 L
1.25 Kg	5.63 L	630 ml	6.25 L
1.50 Kg	6.75 L	750 ml	7.50 L
1.75 Kg	7.88 L	880 ml	8.75 L
2.00 Kg	9.00 L	1.00 L	10.00 L
2.50 Kg	11.25 L	1.25 L	12.50 L
3.00 Kg	13.50 L	1.50 L	15.00 L

1:4 90% (Ethanol)   Dried Herb

Dried Herb	Ethanol	Added water	Total Menstruum
50 g	180 ml	20 ml	200 ml
100 g	360 ml	40 ml	400 ml
150 g	540 ml	60 ml	600 ml
200 g	720 ml	80 ml	800 ml
250 g	900 ml	100 ml	1.00 L
300 g	1.08 L	120 ml	1.20 L
400 g	1.44 L	160 ml	1.60 L
500 g	1.80 L	200 ml	2.00 L
600 g	2.16 L	240 ml	2.40 L
700 g	2.52 L	280 ml	2.80 L
800 g	2.88 L	320 ml	3.20 L
900 g	3.24 L	360 ml	3.60 L
1.00 Kg	3.60 L	400 ml	4.00 L
1.25 Kg	4.50 L	500 ml	5.00 L
1.50 Kg	5.40 L	600 ml	6.00 L
1.75 Kg	6.30 L	700 ml	7.00 L
2.00 Kg	7.20 L	800 ml	8.00 L
2.50 Kg	9.00 L	1.00 L	10.00 L
3.00 Kg	10.80 L	1.20 L	12.00 L

1:3 90% (Ethanol) Dried Herb

Dried Herb	Ethanol	Added water	Total Menstruum
50 g	135 ml	15 ml	150 ml
100 g	270 ml	30 ml	300 ml
150 g	405 ml	45 ml	450 ml
200 g	540 ml	60 ml	600 ml
250 g	675 ml	75 ml	750 ml
300 g	810 ml	90 ml	900 ml
400 g	1.08 L	120 ml	1.20 L
500 g	1.35 L	150 ml	1.50 L
600 g	1.62 L	180 ml	1.80 L
700 g	1.89 L	210 ml	2.10 L
800 g	2.16 L	240 ml	2.40 L
900 g	2.43 L	270 ml	2.70 L
1.00 Kg	2.70 L	300 ml	3.00 L
1.25 Kg	3.38 L	380 ml	3.75 L
1.50 Kg	4.05 L	450 ml	4.50 L
1.75 Kg	4.73 L	530 ml	5.25 L
2.00 Kg	5.40 L	600 ml	6.00 L
2.50 Kg	6.75 L	750 ml	7.50 L
3.00 Kg	8.10 L	900 ml	9.00 L

1:2 90% (Ethanol)   Dried Herb

Dried Herb	Ethanol	Added water	Total Menstruum
50 g	90 ml	10 ml	100 ml
100 g	180 ml	20 ml	200 ml
150 g	270 ml	30 ml	300 ml
200 g	360 ml	40 ml	400 ml
250 g	450 ml	50 ml	500 ml
300 g	540 ml	60 ml	600 ml
400 g	720 ml	80 ml	800 ml
500 g	900 ml	100 ml	1.00 L
600 g	1.08 L	120 ml	1.20 L
700 g	1.26 L	140 ml	1.40 L
800 g	1.44 L	160 ml	1.60 L
900 g	1.62 L	180 ml	1.80 L
1.00 Kg	1.80 L	200 ml	2.00 L
1.25 Kg	2.25 L	250 ml	2.50 L
1.50 Kg	2.70 L	300 ml	3.00 L
1.75 Kg	3.15 L	350 ml	3.50 L
2.00 Kg	3.60 L	400 ml	4.00 L
2.50 Kg	4.50 L	500 ml	5.00 L
3.00 Kg	5.40 L	600 ml	6.00 L

1:1   90% (Ethanol) F.E.   Dried Herb

Dried Herb	Ethanol	Added water	Total Menstruum
50 g	45 ml	5 ml	50 ml
100 g	90 ml	10 ml	100 ml
150 g	135 ml	15 ml	150 ml
200 g	180 ml	20 ml	200 ml
250 g	225 ml	25 ml	250 ml
300 g	270 ml	30 ml	300 ml
400 g	360 ml	40 ml	400 ml
500 g	450 ml	50 ml	500 ml
600 g	540 ml	60 ml	600 ml
700 g	630 ml	70 ml	700 ml
800 g	720 ml	80 ml	800 ml
900 g	810 ml	90 ml	900 ml
1.00 Kg	900 ml	100 ml	1.00 L
1.25 Kg	1.13 L	130 ml	1.25 L
1.50 Kg	1.35 L	150 ml	1.50 L
1.75 Kg	1.58 L	180 ml	1.75 L
2.00 Kg	1.80 L	200 ml	2.00 L
2.50 Kg	2.25 L	250 ml	2.50 L
3.00 Kg	2.70 L	300 ml	3.00 L

1:5 25% (Ethanol)   Fresh Herb

Fresh Herb	Ethanol	Added water	Total Menstruum
50 g	62 ml	150 ml	250 ml
100 g	125 ml	300 ml	500 ml
150 g	187.5 ml	450 ml	750 ml
200 g	250 ml	600 ml	1.00 L
250 g	312 ml	750 ml	1.25 L
300 g	375 ml	900 ml	1.50 L
400 g	500 ml	1.20 L	2.00 L
500 g	625 ml	1.50 L	2.50 L
600 g	750 ml	1.80 L	3.00 L
700 g	875 ml	2.10 L	3.50 L
800 g	1.00 L	2.40 L	4.00 L
900 g	1.12 L	2.70 L	4.50 L
1.00 Kg	1.25 L	3.00 L	5.00 L
1.25 Kg	1.56 L	3.75 L	6.25 L
1.50 Kg	1.88 L	4.50 L	7.50 L
1.75 Kg	2.19 L	5.25 L	8.75 L
2.00 Kg	2.50 L	6.00 L	10.00 L
2.50 Kg	3.13 L	7.50 L	12.50 L
3.00 Kg	3.75 L	9.00 L	15.00 L

This formula assumes the fresh herb contains 75% water by weight

1:4 25% (Ethanol) Fresh Herb

Fresh Herb	Ethanol	Added water	Total Menstruum
50 g	50 ml	113 ml	200 ml
100 g	100 ml	225 ml	400 ml
150 g	150 ml	338 ml	600 ml
200 g	200 ml	450 ml	800 ml
250 g	250 ml	563 ml	1.00 L
300 g	300 ml	675 ml	1.20 L
400 g	400 ml	900 ml	1.60 L
500 g	500 ml	1.12 L	2.00 L
600 g	600 ml	1.35 L	2.40 L
700 g	700 ml	1.57 L	2.80 L
800 g	800 ml	1.80 L	3.20 L
900 g	900 ml	2.02 L	3.60 L
1.00 Kg	1.00 L	2.25 L	4.00 L
1.25 Kg	1.25 L	2.81 L	5.00 L
1.50 Kg	1.50 L	3.38 L	6.00 L
1.75 Kg	1.75 L	3.94 L	7.00 L
2.00 Kg	2.00 L	4.50 L	8.00 L
2.50 Kg	2.50 L	5.63 L	10.00 L
3.00 Kg	3.00 L	6.75 L	12.00 L

This formula assumes the fresh herb contains 75% water by weight

1:3 25% (Ethanol) Fresh Herb

Fresh Herb	Ethanol	Added water	Total Menstruum
50 g	37 ml	75 ml	150 ml
100 g	75 ml	150 ml	300 ml
150 g	112 ml	225 ml	450 ml
200 g	150 ml	300 ml	600 ml
250 g	187 ml	375 ml	750 ml
300 g	225 ml	450 ml	900 ml
400 g	300 ml	600 ml	1.20 L
500 g	375 ml	750 ml	1.50 L
600 g	450 ml	900 ml	1.80 L
700 g	525 ml	1.05 L	2.10 L
800 g	600 ml	1.20 L	2.40 L
900 g	675 ml	1.35 L	2.70 L
1.00 Kg	750 ml	1.50 L	3.00 L
1.25 Kg	940 ml	1.88 L	3.75 L
1.50 Kg	1.13 L	2.25 L	4.50 L
1.75 Kg	1.31 L	2.63 L	5.25 L
2.00 Kg	1.50 L	3.00 L	6.00 L
2.50 Kg	1.88 L	3.75 L	7.50 L
3.00 Kg	2.25 L	4.50 L	9.00 L

This formula assumes the fresh herb contains 75% water by weight

1:2 25% (Ethanol)   Fresh Herb

Fresh Herb	Ethanol	Added water	Total Menstruum
50 g	25 ml	38 ml	100 ml
100 g	50 ml	75 ml	200 ml
150 g	75 ml	113 ml	300 ml
200 g	100 ml	150 ml	400 ml
250 g	125 ml	188 ml	500 ml
300 g	150 ml	225 ml	600 ml
400 g	200 ml	300 ml	800 ml
500 g	250 ml	375 ml	1.00 L
600 g	300 ml	450 ml	1.20 L
700 g	350 ml	525 ml	1.40 L
800 g	400 ml	600 ml	1.60 L
900 g	450 ml	675 ml	1.80 L
1.00 Kg	500 ml	750 ml	2.00 L
1.25 Kg	630 ml	940 ml	2.50 L
1.50 Kg	750 ml	1.13 L	3.00 L
1.75 Kg	880 ml	1.31 L	3.50 L
2.00 Kg	1.00 L	1.50 L	4.00 L
2.50 Kg	1.25 L	1.88 L	5.00 L
3.00 Kg	1.50 L	2.25 L	6.00 L

This formula assumes the fresh herb contains 75% water by weight

1:1   25%   (Ethanol) F.E   Fresh Herb

Fresh Herb	Ethanol	Added water	Total Menstruum
50 g	13 ml	0 ml	50 ml
100 g	25 ml	0 ml	100 ml
150 g	38 ml	0 ml	150 ml
200 g	50 ml	0 ml	200 ml
250 g	63 ml	0 ml	250 ml
300 g	75 ml	0 ml	300 ml
400 g	100 ml	0 ml	400 ml
500 g	125 ml	0 ml	500 ml
600 g	150 ml	0 ml	600 ml
700 g	175 ml	0 ml	700 ml
800 g	200 ml	0 ml	800 ml
900 g	225 ml	0 ml	900 ml
1.00 Kg	250 ml	0.00 L	1.00 L
1.25 Kg	310 ml	0.00 L	1.25 L
1.50 Kg	380 ml	0.00 L	1.50 L
1.75 Kg	440 ml	0.00 L	1.75 L
2.00 Kg	500 ml	0.00 L	2.00 L
2.50 Kg	630 ml	0.00 L	2.50 L
3.00 Kg	750 ml	0.00 L	3.00 L

This formula assumes the fresh herb contains 75% water by weight

1:5   35% (Ethanol)   Fresh Herb

Fresh Herb	Ethanol	Added water	Total Menstruum
50 g	88 ml	125 ml	250 ml
100 g	175 ml	250 ml	500 ml
150 g	263 ml	375 ml	750 ml
200 g	350 ml	500 ml	1.00 L
250 g	438 ml	625 ml	1.25 L
300 g	525 ml	750 ml	1.50 L
400 g	700 ml	1.00 L	2.00 L
500 g	875 ml	1.25 L	2.50 L
600 g	1.05 L	1.50 L	3.00 L
700 g	1.22 L	1.75 L	3.50 L
800 g	1.40 L	2.00 L	4.00 L
900 g	1.57 L	2.25 L	4.50 L
1.00 Kg	1.75 L	2.50 L	5.00 L
1.25 Kg	2.19 L	3.13 L	6.25 L
1.50 Kg	2.63 L	3.75 L	7.50 L
1.75 Kg	3.06 L	4.38 L	8.75 L
2.00 Kg	3.50 L	5.00 L	10.00 L
2.50 Kg	4.38 L	6.25 L	12.50 L
3.00 Kg	5.25 L	7.50 L	15.00 L

This formula assumes the fresh herb contains 75% water by weight

1:4 35% (Ethanol)   Fresh Herb

Fresh Herb	Ethanol	Added water	Total Menstruum
50 g	70 ml	93 ml	200 ml
100 g	140 ml	185 ml	400 ml
150 g	210 ml	278 ml	600 ml
200 g	280 ml	370 ml	800 ml
250 g	350 ml	463 ml	1.00 L
300 g	420 ml	555 ml	1.20 L
400 g	560 ml	740 ml	1.60 L
500 g	700 ml	925 ml	2.00 L
600 g	840 ml	1.11 L	2.40 L
700 g	980 ml	1.29 L	2.80 L
800 g	1.12 L	1.48 L	3.20 L
900 g	1.26 L	1.66 L	3.60 L
1.00 Kg	1.40 L	1.85 L	4.00 L
1.25 Kg	1.75 L	2.31 L	5.00 L
1.50 Kg	2.10 L	2.78 L	6.00 L
1.75 Kg	2.45 L	3.24 L	7.00 L
2.00 Kg	2.80 L	3.70 L	8.00 L
2.50 Kg	3.50 L	4.63 L	10.00 L
3.00 Kg	4.20 L	5.55 L	12.00 L

This formula assumes the fresh herb contains 75% water by weight

1:3 35% (Ethanol) Fresh Herb

Fresh Herb	Ethanol	Added water	Total Menstruum
50 g	53 ml	60 ml	150 ml
100 g	105 ml	120 ml	300 ml
150 g	158 ml	180 ml	450 ml
200 g	210 ml	240 ml	600 ml
250 g	263 ml	300 ml	750 ml
300 g	315 ml	360 ml	900 ml
400 g	420 ml	480 ml	1.20 L
500 g	525 ml	600 ml	1.50 L
600 g	630 ml	720 ml	1.80 L
700 g	735 ml	840 ml	2.10 L
800 g	840 ml	960 ml	2.40 L
900 g	945 ml	1.08 L	2.70 L
1.00 Kg	1.05 L	1.20 L	3.00 L
1.25 Kg	1.31 L	1.50 L	3.75 L
1.50 Kg	1.58 L	1.80 L	4.50 L
1.75 Kg	1.84 L	2.10 L	5.25 L
2.00 Kg	2.10 L	2.40 L	6.00 L
2.50 Kg	2.63 L	3.00 L	7.50 L
3.00 Kg	3.15 L	3.60 L	9.00 L

This formula assumes the fresh herb contains 75% water by weight

1:2 35% (Ethanol) Fresh Herb

Fresh Herb	Ethanol	Added water	Total Menstruum
50 g	35 ml	28 ml	100 ml
100 g	70 ml	55 ml	200 ml
150 g	105 ml	83 ml	300 ml
200 g	140 ml	110 ml	400 ml
250 g	175 ml	138 ml	500 ml
300 g	210 ml	165 ml	600 ml
400 g	280 ml	220 ml	800 ml
500 g	350 ml	275 ml	1.00 L
600 g	420 ml	330 ml	1.20 L
700 g	490 ml	385 ml	1.40 L
800 g	560 ml	440 ml	1.60 L
900 g	630 ml	495 ml	1.80 L
1.00 Kg	700 ml	0.55 L	2.00 L
1.25 Kg	880 ml	0.69 L	2.50 L
1.50 Kg	1.05 L	0.83 L	3.00 L
1.75 Kg	1.23 L	0.96 L	3.50 L
2.00 Kg	1.40 L	1.10 L	4.00 L
2.50 Kg	1.75 L	1.38 L	5.00 L
3.00 Kg	2.10 L	1.65 L	6.00 L

This formula assumes the fresh herb contains 75% water by weight

1:5   45% (Ethanol)   Fresh Herb

Fresh Herb	Ethanol	Added water	Total Menstruum
50 g	113 ml	100 ml	250 ml
100 g	225 ml	200 ml	500 ml
150 g	338 ml	300 ml	750 ml
200 g	450 ml	400 ml	1.00 L
250 g	563 ml	500 ml	1.25 L
300 g	675 ml	600 ml	1.50 L
400 g	900 ml	800 ml	2.00 L
500 g	1.12 L	1.00 L	2.50 L
600 g	1.35 L	1.20 L	3.00 L
700 g	1.57 L	1.40 L	3.50 L
800 g	1.80 L	1.60 L	4.00 L
900 g	2.02 L	1.80 L	4.50 L
1.00 Kg	2.25 L	2.00 L	5.00 L
1.25 Kg	2.81 L	2.50 L	6.25 L
1.50 Kg	3.38 L	3.00 L	7.50 L
1.75 Kg	3.94 L	3.50 L	8.75 L
2.00 Kg	4.50 L	4.00 L	10.00 L
2.50 Kg	5.63 L	5.00 L	12.50 L
3.00 Kg	6.75 L	6.00 L	15.00 L

This formula assumes the fresh herb contains 75% water by weight

1:4 45% (Ethanol)   Fresh Herb

Fresh Herb	Ethanol	Added water	Total Menstruum
50 g	90 ml	73 ml	200 ml
100 g	180 ml	145 ml	400 ml
150 g	270 ml	218 ml	600 ml
200 g	360 ml	290 ml	800 ml
250 g	450 ml	363 ml	1.00 L
300 g	540 ml	435 ml	1.20 L
400 g	720 ml	580 ml	1.60 L
500 g	900 ml	725 ml	2.00 L
600 g	1.08 L	870 ml	2.40 L
700 g	1.26 L	1015 ml	2.80 L
800 g	1.44 L	1160 ml	3.20 L
900 g	1.62 L	1305 ml	3.60 L
1.00 Kg	1.80 L	1.45 L	4.00 L
1.25 Kg	2.25 L	1.81 L	5.00 L
1.50 Kg	2.70 L	2.18 L	6.00 L
1.75 Kg	3.15 L	2.54 L	7.00 L
2.00 Kg	3.60 L	2.90 L	8.00 L
2.50 Kg	4.50 L	3.63 L	10.00 L
3.00 Kg	5.40 L	4.35 L	12.00 L

This formula assumes the fresh herb contains 75% water by weight

1:3 45% (Ethanol)   Fresh Herb

Fresh Herb	Ethanol	Added water	Total Menstruum
50 g	68 ml	45 ml	150 ml
100 g	135 ml	90 ml	300 ml
150 g	203 ml	135 ml	450 ml
200 g	270 ml	180 ml	600 ml
250 g	338 ml	225 ml	750 ml
300 g	405 ml	270 ml	900 ml
400 g	540 ml	360 ml	1200 ml
500 g	675 ml	450 ml	1500 ml
600 g	810 ml	540 ml	1800 ml
700 g	945 ml	630 ml	2100 ml
800 g	1080 ml	720 ml	2400 ml
900 g	1215 ml	810 ml	2700 ml
1.00 Kg	1.35 L	0.90 L	3.00 L
1.25 Kg	1.69 L	1.13 L	3.75 L
1.50 Kg	2.03 L	1.35 L	4.50 L
1.75 Kg	2.36 L	1.58 L	5.25 L
2.00 Kg	2.70 L	1.80 L	6.00 L
2.50 Kg	3.38 L	2.25 L	7.50 L
3.00 Kg	4.05 L	2.70 L	9.00 L

This formula assumes the fresh herb contains 75% water by weight

1:2 45% (Ethanol) — Fresh Herb

Fresh Herb	Ethanol	Added water	Total Menstruum
50 g	45 ml	18 ml	100 ml
100 g	90 ml	35 ml	200 ml
150 g	135 ml	53 ml	300 ml
200 g	180 ml	70 ml	400 ml
250 g	225 ml	88 ml	500 ml
300 g	270 ml	105 ml	600 ml
400 g	360 ml	140 ml	800 ml
500 g	450 ml	175 ml	1.00 L
600 g	540 ml	210 ml	1.20 L
700 g	630 ml	245 ml	1.40 L
800 g	720 ml	280 ml	1.60 L
900 g	810 ml	315 ml	1.80 L
1.00 Kg	900 ml	350 ml	2.00 L
1.25 Kg	1.13 L	440 ml	2.50 L
1.50 Kg	1.35 L	530 ml	3.00 L
1.75 Kg	1.58 L	610 ml	3.50 L
2.00 Kg	1.80 L	700 ml	4.00 L
2.50 Kg	2.25 L	880 ml	5.00 L
3.00 Kg	2.70 L	1.05 L	6.00 L

This formula assumes the fresh herb contains 75% water by weight

Part 4

Appendices:

Further Reading

Schedule III/20 Tincture Specs

Western Herbal Medicine has access to some quite strong herbs. These are potentially poisonous herbs and are controlled in the UK (and possibly other countries too). Such herbs are listed in what used to be called Schedule III of the medicines act, 1968, superceded by Schedule 20 of the Human Medicines Regulation 2012.

Schedule III
or
Part 2 Poison

For those wishing to make their own Schedule III/20 tinctures here is a table of specifications, adapted from the catalogues of four UK herbal tincture suppliers.

Herb Name	Tincture Spec.	F.E. Spec.
Ammi visnaga	1:3 45%	1:1 45%
Arnica montana	1:10 45%, 1:8 35%	1:1 45%
Atropa beladonna fol.	1:10 45%	
Chelidonium majus	1:5 45%, 1:5 35%	1:1 45%
Convallaria majalis	1:5 45%1:5 25%	
Datura stratammonium	1:10 45%	
Ephedra sinica	1:5 45%, 1:5 25%	1:1 45%
Gelsemium sempervirens	1:10 45%, 1:10 60%	
Hyoscymus niger	1:10 45%	
Lobelia inflata	1:5 45%	

The (UK) Law on Tincture Making

The law is a complicated and convoluted subject that the following is not intended to be canonical fact or legal advice, it is simply the author's understanding of what is allowed as it currently stands.

Unless you have a licence to receive duty free spirits, you are stuck with buying vodka, or buying 96% grain spirit upon which you must pay duty at an exorbitant rate. A licence to receive duty free spirits can be obtained free of charge from HMRC (See suppliers). DFS must be kept in a locked area away from the public. When you apply for your licence, you will need to send a complete list of herbs you intend to make into tinctures (Copy from one of the larger catalogues) to HMRC, along with a drawing of where you intend to keep your DFS. You *will* be told that something on your list is prohibited and there seems to be little reason for what the official rubber-stamping your application will decide to prohibit on the day he grants your licence.

Anyone is free to make tinctures, however, following GMP (Good Manufacturing Practice) is advisable, especially if the tinctures will be offered for sale, though it is likely that some smaller tincture makers do not follow GMP.

Selling tinctures to the public as medicinal products without a THMP licence is forbidden, though some tinctures that could be considered food extracts could be sold as such if clearly labeled as a food product for non-medicinal use (i.e. vanilla tincture sold as flavouring in cooking falls under this heading). However, this may class the tinctures as beverages requiring an alcohol licence to sell; a condition for the manufacture and sale of these tinctures using duty free spirits is that they be sold 'presented as a medicinal product'

Anyone can sell tinctures to other herbalists (which isn't a defined title/qualification in law) as long as the conditions of sale are that they are '*For administration under section 12(1) of the medicines act 1968*' and that bottles are clearly labeled as such.

There is EU legislation on the requirements for pharmaceutical ingredients - i.e. tinctures sold to herbalists. This includes required GMP. This legislation is covered in: Council Directive 2008/4/EC: European Commission – The Rules Governing Medicine Products in the European Union – Volume 4 – Annex 7 – 1st September 2008

You are strongly advised to look up the Medicines Act 1968, The Human Medicines Regulations 2012, and the Licensing Act 2003, read them and make your own mind up - or take legal advice in order to do so!

Further Reading

For anyone wanting to read a more general overview of herbal medicine making, I have found the following books to be most invaluable; they come strongly recommended.

The Herbal Medicine Maker's Handbook: A Home Manual.
James Green, 2000.
ISBN: 978-0895949905

Modern Herbal Dispensatory: A Medicine-Making Guide
Thomas Easley & Steven Horne, 2017.
ISBN: 978-1623170790

Hedgerow Medicine: Harvest and Make Your Own Herbal Remedies
Julie Bruton-Seal &Matthew Seal, 2008.
ISBN: 978-1873674994

Transcript & Notes from a pharmacy workshop including information on setting up an Alembic still:

http://tiny.cc/alembicsetup

Suppliers

Bulk Herbs

Organic Herb Trading Company

Butts Way, Milverton, TA4 1ND
01823 401205   http://www.organicherbtrading.com/

Grain Spirit

Haymankimia

70 Eastways, Witham, CM8 3YE
01376 517517   http://www.haymankimia.co.uk/

Joseph Mills Denaturants Ltd.

0151 421 0014   https://www.ethanol.co.uk/

Tincture Presses

Vigo Presses Ltd.

4 Flightway, Dunkeswell, Honiton, EX14 4RD
01404 890093   http://www.vigopresses.co.uk/

Alembic Stills

Potz Copper

101E Victoria Drive, London, SW19 6PT
                    https://www.potzcopper.co.uk/

Percolators

Byron Botanicals (Australia)

+61 0401 883 700   http://byronbotanicals.com.au/

Licence to receive Duty Free Spirits

Her Majesty's Revenue & Customs (HMRC)

Excise Written Enquiries Team, Ground Floor, Portcullis House, 21 India Street Glasgow G2 4PZ

0300 200 3700   https://www.gov.uk/hmrc

Glossary

Alcohol	= any organic compound in which the hydroxyl functional group is bound to a saturated carbon atom. Often used as a synonym for Ethanol.
Amphipathic	= Dissolves both oil and water.
Decoction	= The concentrated liquor resulting from heating or boiling a substance, especially a medicinal preparation made from a plant.
Distillation	= the process of separating or concentrating volatile constituents or substances from a liquid mixture by selective evaporation and condensation.
Ethanol	= A 2-carbom alcohol used in incture making and alcoholic beverages. Formula: C_2H_5OH.
Glycerite	= A liquid extract using glycerine, (a sugar alcohol) as the solvent.
Grain Spirit	= a 96% ABV azeotrope of ethanol and water made from fermenting and distilling grain

Infusion	= extract prepared by soaking leaves or herbs in liquid, usually boiling water
Maceration	= Preparation of an extract by solvent extraction, usually soaking.
Marc	= The herbal material used (often macerated) in tincturemaking.
Menstruum	= The liquid used in tincture making, specifically that which is pressed out of the *marc* at the end of the tincturemaking process.
Percolation	= The process of a liquid slowly passing through a filter, in the case of tincturemaking the filter is a bed of plant material.
Spec.	= Abbr. Specification. The information on how a tincture was prepared: its strength, alcohol content and extraction method.
Still	= A device for extracting concentrated volatile compounds. In the herbal world usually refers to some kind of retort: a pot still or alembic.
Tincture	= An alcoholic extract.

Measurement Conversion Table

Weights - Metric

1 Litre (L)   = 1000 Millilitres (ml)

1 Kilogram (Kg) = 1000 Grams (g)

Densities *

Water: 1 ml = 1g

Ethanol: 1 ml = .78g

* At room temperature, normal atmospheric pressure

US Imperial - Metric - US Imperial

Proof = % Alcohol by Vol x 2 - % Alcohol by vol = Proof ÷ 2

US Fl. Oz. = 29.57 ml   -   30 ml = 1.01 US Fl. Oz

US Oz.   = 28.34 g   -   30 g = 1.05 US Oz.

US Cup   = 236.5 ml   -   236.5 ml = 1 US Cup.

US Pt.   = 0.47 L   =   1 L   = 2.11 US Pt.

US Lb.   = 0.45 Kg   -   1 Kg = 2.20 US Lb.

www.ingramcontent.com/pod-product-compliance
Lightning Source LLC
Chambersburg PA
CBHW070303230526
45470CB00002B/699